Weight Loss & Fitness Myths Debunked for Rookies

Mirsad Hasic

DEDICATION

I dedicate this book to my wife.

CONTENTS

1   Getting Older Means Getting Fatter   1

2   Crash Dieting Works Well   Pg 4

3   Is Exercising Early in The Day The Most Effective   Pg 8

4   The Lie of TV-Shop Machines   Pg 11

5   Don't Eat After 8 P.M   Pg 15

6   Do Not Avoid Carbohydrates   Pg 18

7   Spot Reducing Bely Fat   Pg 21

8   Genes Determines Your Weight Loss   Pg 24

9   Fat is Really Harmful to Health. Isn't it?   Pg 27

10 Vegetarian Diets are Better for Losing Weight   Pg 30

11 Products Labeled as 'Zero Trans-Fat'   Pg 33

12 Dairy Products Makes You Fat   Pg 36

13 Eggs Raise The Bad Cholesterol Levels   Pg 39

14 Bananas Are Fattening   Pg 42

15 Nuts Make You Fat!   Pg 45

16 You Should Avoid Meat   Pg 48

17 Lifting Weights Will Bulk You up   Pg 51

18 Skip a Meal or Two & Lose Weight   Pg 54

ACKNOWLEDGMENTS

I would like to thank my family for their support.

1. GETTING OLDER MEANS GETTING FATTER

Myth: The older you get the more weight you'll put on, thus having a big belly is justified!

This topic is something I often debate with my father, who is presently overweight. He tries to convince me that the older I become, the more pounds I will pile on.

Of course, he makes sure to remind me that it's out of my control. He says that as you age and your metabolism slows down, so the force of nature takes over, and that's all there is to it!

Fact: I always respond to this by saying it's simply not true. Okay, so we all know that the ability to gain muscles decreases the older we get, but that still doesn't mean we can justify being overweight just because of a loss in muscle mass.

According to a study published in the International Journal of Obesity by Dr. PT Williams, he states that older people don't gain weight because of their age per se.

The research suggests there are three other factors that are responsible for this problem:

1. A greater intake of calories at a time when the body's metabolism is decreasing
2. A more sedentary lifestyle which increases the amount of fat stored
3. Little or no exercise using weights, thus decreasing muscle mass. [1]

My experience is that the older people become, the harder they are to convince about the real health dangers associated with being overweight or obese.

A lot of older folks can't actually see why they should start working out when they have been living, and perhaps even enjoying, an inactive lifestyle for a good many years.

In other words, the mere thought of seriously exercising at middle-age, and older, doesn't exactly seem inviting for most. The majority would rather stay at home, put their feet up, and just drink and eat whatever they want when they want to.

They probably think they've earned it, but the reality is that inactivity and an unhealthy diet can, and often does, send many people to an early grave.

What we should all be mindful of is that age is only a number, and it doesn't mean we should just sit back and watch ourselves wither away

I've meet seniors who were able to lift more on the bench press than most of the younger guys at the gym. I've also competed against seniors during running competitions that were completely outstanding, and I do mean exceptional.

Physical exercise is really something we ought to be doing throughout our entire life, as well as eating a nutritious diet. Even so, there are still huge benefits to be had from adopting a healthy lifestyle change at any age, so all is not lost.

You need to ask yourself how long you want to live for, and that means 'living' not just 'existing'. With each new generation we see life expectancy rise, but sadly, it usually just means people are sicker for longer, thanks, or not, to modern medicine. If you want to live for as long as you can while maintaining your health, then keep reading.

Even if you're one of those folks who lives for the 'now' and cares little about your physical condition, you might still want to think of those who would be devastated if you were to depart before your time.

We have a responsibility to our families and loved ones, and by starting to live a more active and healthy life means you guys can get to enjoy each other for longer.

So I really want you to forget everything you know, or think you know, that is thought to be related to age and flab, because it's pure hogwash.

Health experts consider the age and 'inevitable' weight issue as something of a poor excuse used by older folks for letting themselves go then blaming it on the years.

I am aware of the fact that there are some parts to the ageing process that you can't control, but there are many others that you can.

With a little discipline and a genuine desire to change, then looking, feeling, and functioning better, is well within your grasp.

2. CRASH DIETING WORKS WELL

Myth: It's easy to lose several pounds of weight rapidly if you just follow one of the many crash diet properly.

Fact: I am sure that you know this already, but when something sounds too good to be true, then it usually is. Furthermore, most of these rapid weight loss programs don't even come close to what they promise.

In many cases, crash dieting, or starvation diets as they're sometimes referred to, do little more than dehydrate the dieter, and that means the lost weight is little more than water. Needless to say, it is gained back as fast as it was lost once the regime ends.

Let's not forget too that when someone goes ON a diet, it means they will likely come OFF it as soon as the target weight is reached. But to maintain a healthy weight means making lifestyle changes, and not going on some sort of intense course.

Take crash dieting for example. This could never be sustainable as a lifestyle change. It might lose you a few pounds (of water mainly), and you will become a little slimmer, but most of the fat is still there, latent, and waiting to spread out again the moment you become properly rehydrated. Even if that sounds okay for those folks wanting to shed a few pounds before a holiday, or some important event perhaps, there are still some things you should know about these kinds of diets.

The crash diet is one of the worst and most dangerous ways of losing weight period. In fact, it can cause direct harm to your body and affect your mood.

Yet despite all of this, these potentially dangerous eating plans are still legally promoted all over the place, preying on the vulnerable.

In my experience, most weightwatchers who have tried to fight the flab have attempted the rapid dieting method at least once. But I also know people who go on these starvation plans regularly, and that's just asking for trouble since it's dangerous for the heart!

Isadore Rosenfeld, MD, a professor in clinical medicine, states that trying a crash diet once won't necessary harm your heart or your overall health.

But if you make it into a habit then you are putting yourself at risk, as the chance of heart attack increases each time you go on these super-fast weight loss programs!

Each time I hear someone shouting from the rooftops on how they lost ten pounds in one week, I raise my eyebrows and look at them somewhat skeptically.

Sure, they might have achieved this, but remember that 75% of our body is made up of water, and most of this rapid weight loss would have been exactly that - water [2]!

There's little point in losing water weight if the fat still remains. The first thing that happens with a crash diets is that you're getting rid of muscle mass, not fat, and less muscle means more fat.

The consequence of this is if you lose too much muscle you will also reduce your chance of losing weight.

I don't know how many times I've tried to make people understand that crash dieting is one of the worst possible methods they can use for weight loss.

Alas, what I explain all too often falls on deaf ears. Usually, I get a response like this:

"Mirsad, so what you are telling me is that crash dieting doesn't work, right? If that's true, how come each morning when I step onto the scales I see a lower number? I'm either lighter or I'm not, and the scales never lie!"

It doesn't seem to matter how many times I try to explain this lower number is mostly a loss in water. I tell them that the moment they come off their diet and start hydrating and eating regularly again, the weight will come back as fast, if not faster than it went.

In many cases, when people come off a crash diet, they will actually gain an extra pound or two, which kind of defeats the purpose.

Another danger with fast weight-loss plans - when done too often - is the potential risk of organ damage. They can become stressed and inflamed, which in turn can make you more receptive to disease and more vulnerable to illnesses and catching viruses in general. Moreover, fast dieting can negatively affect the way you feel and function as a person.

You should also know that people who adopt crash diets not only have the potential to gain extra weight after they stop following this madness, but they are left with an insatiable craving for their old and often unhealthy meals, consisting mainly of fattening and processed foods, which are also damaging to health! Just think of it like this:

Poor diet + Crash diet + Poor diet = long-term health and weight problems.

I understand that the moment a person has decided to do something about their weight once and for all they want quick results, and the faster the better.

I also know that most folks want to get rid of these pounds with the least amount of discomfort and effort. It's important to recognize though that there is no magic solution or quick fixes; this is not how it works.

All those whacky claims out there promising as much are pure baloney. Having said all of that, losing weight does not have to be a lesson in torcher either, providing the dieter approaches it with the right mindset.

So if you can accept that you will need to put the work in (that includes raising a bit of sweat), then you will have a much better chance of keeping a controlled and healthy weight, as opposed to gaining more pounds and health risks with each passing year.

3. IS EXERCISING EARLY IN THE DAY THE MOST EFFECTIVE

Myth: If you want to lose as much weight as possible you should exercise in the mornings!

Fact: Honestly, I don't know how many times I've heard my friends and relatives go on about how effectual it is to exercise early in the morning, convinced that it's the best way to accelerate maximum weight loss.

I've even been forced by my wife to get up early during the weekends because some self-proclaimed guru at her place of work told her that she could burn off more fat by exercising at sunrise.

Although there are studies claiming that you get better results by working out early in the day, I decided to dig into this myth and do a bit of research myself in order to form my own opinion.

I gathered together various books and scientific publications, all of which were written by those with real authority on the subject, and not just by one of the plethora of self-confessed health and fitness gurus who blog on the internet.

Needless to say, I was not surprised when I found studies that stated the best time to exercise is actually when you feel like it, or are most motivated.

Very few people are totally pumped up and ready roll at the crack of dawn, and that means the majority won't perform at their best, unless of course it really is a time when they want to, and not simply feel like they have to.

This is a proven fact, and Samantha B. Cassetty M.S., R.D., from the Good Housekeeping Research Institute, says that best time to do your exercise is anytime you have the time, and let's face it, when we do have time, we're genuinely more motivated and enthusiastic anyway [3].

Early morning exercise is not only impractical for most family people, but can actually add stress to the mornings; something that's quite unhealthy by itself.

Let's say you have two kids that you need to get ready for the kindergarten, and then you have a 30 minute drive into work.

Personally I don't know how anyone could relish the thought of waking up, working out, showering, preparing and eating breakfast, taking care of the kids, and all the other start of day procedures many of today's busy families have to do soon after the alarm goes off. Whoever said that early morning is the best time to exercise got that totally wrong in my opinion.

It's hardly surprising that so many people who begin their fitness regime at dawn quickly become burned out and demotivated, and so end up giving up shortly after they started.

While I admire people who are able to get up at 5:00 a.m. to walk or run in the dark while the snow is falling (we have seven months of winter here in Sweden), I can't really see why I would want to force myself to do it.

Remember, there's a huge difference between wanting to exercise at daybreak and feeling you need to, and I hope by reading here

I've managed to convince you that it's not necessary, not at all.

However, while you might not be able to lose more weight by exercising in the morning, there have been studies that suggest it can improve the quality of your sleep.

Getting a good night's kip is a highly important factor when it comes to losing weight, so I'm not totally dismissing early morning workouts as a negative thing, but merely pointing out the fact that they do not assist weight loss.

A study performed by Driver & Taylor at the Department of Psychiatry, University of Toronto, showed that exercising in the mornings can improve the quality of sleep, while exercising in the evenings could actually have the opposite effect in some folks, especially if they train too close to bedtime.

So if you are someone who has problems with sleep, then you might want to consider the early morning workout. If you sleep like a baby, and don't like to physically train at dawn, then you really don't have to. [4]

To summarize then (based on the scientific studies I've found), working out early is not going to burn off more weight than at any other time of day.

Instead, it's better to workout whenever you have time to commit to a good session. Exercising when you want to, rather than when you believed you had to, is going to deliver the best all round results.

4. THE LIE OF TV-SHOP MACHINES

Myth: The machines advertised on the late TV commercials work incredibly well, and by using them, you too can get the same body as the models demonstrating these machines!

Fact: This is one of the oldest lies when it comes to losing weight from the comfort of home.

I bet that even if you have never purchased a home gym (or other exercise device designed specifically for home use), from these shopping channels, you have at least been tempted to do so once or twice, am I right?

Usually they bring in a few models, obviously with great looking bodies, that do some peculiar and often new kinds of exercises, which are claimed to be revolutionary.

Viewers become enticed to order while stocks or promotions last, and hope that their purchase will help them get that well defined body in record time.

But even if they did work, it's a proven fact that 40 percent of people who invest in home exercise machines barely use them after just a few days or weeks.

The reason why these machines are constantly being promoted over and over is because people continue to get sucked in by the hype and buy them. I know this sounds cliché, but there isn't an exercise machine out there that can help anyone lose weight by using it for just five minutes a day; the crazy claims made by some manufacturers and retailers.

The problem with people in general is that we humans have become physically lazy by nature. This means we're constantly on the lookout for anything that will give us the body we so desire, and with a minimum amount of effort.

But this wishful thinking only makes us vulnerable, and that is why we tend to continually buy into such wild claims made by those selling these exercise machines. Despite all the hype, the miracle fat-busting apparatus hasn't been invented yet, and probably never will.

One example of how these things are promoted is a product that was claimed to 'spot reduce' belly fat. It was frequently advertised as the AB Energizer Exercise System. What it is, is a simple belt that you attach to your belly, push the power button, and voila!

You should be able to watch the magic happen as the belt burns away your fat so that you don't have to. What a fallacy that turned out to be!

One friend of mine, who is actually quite a smart guy in most areas of life, was unlucky enough to fall for this commercial, and purchased the belt for $100. A few days later it arrived in the mailbox, and he was really excited about using it.

After just three minutes of use the batteries died, and the only thing he got was a few beads of sweat around his belly area. He went to the store and purchased ten batteries that cost him around $30.

After using the belt for 30 minutes the batteries died once again, and he could see that he'd not lost a single ounce of belly fat! By now, it was blatantly apparent that he'd been cheated, and had bought into a scam.

There was a refund policy, but only if the product had not been used or was damaged in some way. But as it was obvious that he'd taken it out of the box and used it, he was stuck with the worthless device.

I can remember how much I laughed when he told me about this, and I still rib him about it to this day. By the way, I did some research on this product and was not surprised when I found out that it has been pulled off the market by the Federal Trade Commission.

Still, that doesn't mean there aren't many other such 'miracle' exercise machines out there preying on the vulnerable, because there are. [5]

And as for my friend, one year later he had totally lost his belly fat and even got a six pack abs, but it wasn't with any kind of revolutionary machine. What he did was make some lifestyle changes, and that meant eating good nutritious foods, and exercising regularly. Eating well, and getting more physical exercise is a simple formula that works very well, but only when we work it!

The lazier we become as a race, the less physical exertion we're prepared to do, and that's sad. Ask anyone who works out and watches what they eat, and they will surely tell you they feel fantastic.

Yet despite it all, there are still so many of us who want a quick outcome, and continue to look for machines which promise fast results – and for next to no effort! I'm guessing that by reading this book, you are not one of them, or are least ready to make some positive changes.

I really want you to learn a lesson from my friend and save your hard earned money for something more worthy.

I guarantee that even if you had an entire roomful of these so called miracle machines - frequently marketed through the infomercials - you would still not get the result they claim or that you desire.

You have most probably heard the expression: "you get out of life what you put into it".

Well, losing weight and maintaining your health levels is no different. In order for you to reach your weight loss goals, you will need to put in the work, and probably make some adjustments to your diet at the same time.

The choice is yours.

Ask yourself if you are now ready to put in the effort required and make some positive adjustments to your lifestyle, or whether you're going to continue watching these TV Ads hoping against hope that the 'revolutionary' fat-burning dream machine is just around the corner?

5. DON'T EAT AFTER 8 P.M.

Myth: If you eat after 8 p.m. you should not expect to lose weight because eating late is what makes you gain those extra pounds!

Fact: I am sure some self-proclaimed fitness guru has said to you that eating after 8pm is a bad idea, and that all the food you consume after this time is actually going to convert into fat and stick to the inside of your body like super glue.

You will be pleased to know that such a claim is pure poppycock. It's not so much when you eat, but what you eat. For example, eating junk food is equally bad no matter whether it's 2 p.m. after a late night out, or as a lunch.

Eating poor quality food (anything that lacks nutrition), late at night, might affect your quality of sleep depending what you consume, how much, and how late, but it's got nothing to do with weight gain.

This is confirmed by the Academy of Nutrition and Dietetics, that state it doesn't matter when you eat but what you eat. It further maintains that calories have exactly the same effect on the body no matter what time you are consuming them [6].

Dr. Mehmet Cengiz, from the show Oz, echoes a similar statement, and says it's not the time of the day that makes you gain weight but the amount of calories an individual consumes during the day. Calories don't know what the time is, and that means it doesn't matter when you consume them [7].

I have health conscious friends and relatives who scream with disbelief if you offer them something to eat after 8 p.m. It always makes me frustrated, and I'm forced to put the evidence in front of them in an attempt to debunk this myth that they've bought into.

Alas, many still trust what has been written somewhere by someone, and changing people's beliefs is often easier said than done, even if you confront them with the facts.

It's been my experience that this is a myth which has risen up in modern times.

This is because of the sheer number of new diets that are constantly popping up, each one giving all kinds of different and conflicting advice, and telling the dieter what's right and what's wrong, but without any real hard evidence to back up their statements.

I can say with total honestly that I always eat after 8.p.m. In actual fact, I would say that this is the time of day when I consume the most food, because after dinner I usually eat a whole load of fruit and combine it with a large protein shake.

It's not unusual for me to consume 500 g of wine grapes, two of three apples, plus one or two bananas, and all of this later at night, which can be anywhere between 7 p.m. to 11 p.m.

However, I still consider myself as being someone who is in very good shape, and yes I have a six pack, believe it or not!

If the myth about eating after 8 p.m. was true, then surely by now I would resemble a pot-bellied pig, rather than a well-toned guy in his 30s.

So if I were you, I would first start evaluating what it is you eat, and not worry about the time of the day when you actually consume it (unless it's very late at night and affects your sleep).

After you take a real good look at the foods you consume over the course of a week, or month, the chance is that you will soon discover the main reasons why you are the weight you have become.

To end this chapter, I really do hope that you will not be stubborn in your beliefs like some of my friends. These guys still think that eating after 8 p.m. is a really bad idea, despite the fact that they know I do, and can visibly see the great shape I'm in.

On average, a stomach full of food takes about three hours to empty. So if you're someone who has their last meal early in the evening, and goes to bed late, then you're going to experience hunger pangs at bedtime.

Okay, so we know that losing weight and getting into shape requires some effort and commitment, but that does not mean you have to suffer hunger in order to achieve your goals.

6. DO NOT AVOID CARBOHYDRATES

Myth: Carbohydrates (or carbs), are one of the hidden pitfalls when it comes to losing weight, and why? Because they make you gain extra pounds without even being aware of it!

Fact: With today's media coverage on living healthier, there have been plenty of myths thrown around warning the public to watch out for this, and stay away from that!

One of the most frequent myths is that if you really want to lose weight then you must avoid carbohydrates.

People today are suspicious and scared to eat anything that has 'carbohydrates' on the label. They have come to believe the item will make them gain weight and therefore spoil all their hard work at losing it.

The massive popularity of 'low carbs diets' has come about because dieters have bought into this myth. Every day I read somewhere about how carbohydrates are evil, and anyone serious about losing weight should avoid them at all costs.

I can assure you here and now that avoiding carbohydrates is a really bad dieting strategy. They are in fact one of the fundamental ingredients used by the body for it to function properly, i.e., they give it energy, and a well-functioning body is better able to help you lose weight than one that is not.

Carbohydrates are typically divided into two different types, known as simple and complex, or sugar and starch.

Simple Carbohydrates (simple sugars)

The refined ones include sugars found in fruits, honey, malt products, milk, and vegetables, but also in less nutritious foods like refined sugars (the white sugar we buy at the supermarket), and ice creams etc.

Complex Carbohydrates (starches)

The other type of carbs is the natural unrefined type, known as complex carbohydrates. These include starches which are found in foods such as grain products, i.e., bread, crackers, pasta, rice, some fruits, and leguminous plants.

Both types of carbohydrate contain some foods that are better choices than others, so understanding the good carbs from the bad is what the dieter needs to learn about.

It's probably fair to say that most refined carbohydrates are jam packed with energy but contain very little nutrition, while the majority of unrefined carbs are the much healthier option, and should be included as a part of your healthy diet.

When you eat carbohydrates they are broken down into something called glucose. Glucose is a simple sugar and an important source of energy for the body.

It really is a crucial nutrient that must enter the cells. You might already know that your cells are responsible for keeping your body functioning properly.

For example, your brain needs about 100 grams of glucose per day in order for it to function well. Another use of glucose is that it's an important ingredient for burning body fat.

This is just a very basic outline on the importance of glucose, but should give you some idea of its significance. In short, your body will not work properly without it!

A healthy diet should contain at least 50% of unrefined carbohydrates and the rest should come from protein sources that can be found in fish, chicken, and beef to name but three.

Some good meatless protein choices may include cereals, dairy, eggs, nuts, seeds, and soy products.

Don't forget to include fat as well from Polyunsaturated/Monounsaturated sources.

I understand that the world of carbohydrates can appear confusing to those unfamiliar with the topic. This is mainly because there is a constant supply of 'new data' coming out from so-called scientifically proven studies, many of which report on the negative aspects of carbohydrates in our diets.

One metaphor I like to use when describing carbohydrates is to imagine that they are the cement used for building houses. The rest of the building is protein, fats and other nutrients.

But none of these other ingredients are of any use without carbohydrates, because they must exist in order to hold it together, make it strong, and truly functional.

I hope by now you can see the importance of including 'good carbs' into your daily diet. Carbohydrates are crucial for losing and maintaining weight loss, and if you try to avoid them in your meals, I can guarantee that you are making a big mistake.

So please, don't buy into the myth that carbs are something to be avoided like the plague, because it's just not so!

7. SPOT REDUCING BELLY FAT

Myth: By performing specific exercises like sit ups and other abdominal workouts, you can spot-reduce your belly fat providing you do enough repetitions!

Fact: Usually, the first thing I hear from people who want to lose weight is, "What type of exercises do I need to do in order to shrink my flabby tummy?"

I don't know how many times I have explained that it is not possible to flatten that stomach with abdominal exercise alone, yet, folks just don't seem to get it.

In my experience, this is one of the main reasons why so many people quit training. They somehow buy into the misconception that by doing only ab exercises, day in and day out, they are going to get that six-pack they're striving for.

In all of such cases the individual ends up disappointed. It's just impossible to reduce fat on a specific area of the body. If we could do it, then all the gyms around the world would shut down because people would never need visit them!

A health and fitness regime is something that includes a number of different exercises, some for building muscle, and others for losing weight and increasing stamina.

To give you a real world example, I will tell you about a friend of mine who was overweight and desperate to get a flat stomach.

Each winter he would say to me, "Mirsad, this is it, this summer I will have that perfect flat stomach, and this time I mean it, I will not fail" And he did mean it, and he was determined, yet still he failed, year in and year out, for five long years.

His problem was that he thought he knew best. Despite me having told the guy a zillion times over that spot reducing fat is impossible, still he chose to ignore my advice and kept looking for that secret formula that would prove me wrong.

Every week he'd find some newfangled exercise gadget, or type of training that would burn his belly fat and give him those six-pack abs he dreamt about. Alas, each time he came away disappointed at how much time, effort, and sometimes money, he lost trying.

And not only did he fail in his attempts to lose the gut, but each year he gained more weight in his pursuit for the 'body beautiful'.

Although I felt really sorry for him, I still wanted to give the guy a good shake and knock some reasoning into him. I tried again and again to explain that the only way to reduce his fat, and flatten that stomach, was to start doing things the right way.

That meant putting together a real exercise regime and eating a healthy diet. In other words, he had to follow through on some lifestyle changes.

Today I don't waste my time because everything I say only falls on deaf ears. He's still overweight and I do feel for him, but he just doesn't want to accept the fact that he can't spot reduce belly fat. So now I just let him get on with things – his way!

If you recognize yourself in my friend here, and perhaps blame anything and everything (other than yourself), for constant failures, then it is really important for you to realize that you CAN NOT spot reduce belly fat.

Anything or anyone who says otherwise is just preaching some mumbo-jumbo hocus-pocus, usually in the form of a product or service that is either spoke of through ignorance, or there's a scam in there somewhere (see chapter 2).

Honestly folks, it takes blood, sweat, and tears to get rid of abdominal fat, and that means focusing on regular training combined with a healthy, nutritious diet. And yes, some sacrifices will have to be made if you're serious about it.

But once your fat stomach becomes flat, maintaining it is less of an effort providing you adhere to the basics. There are no big secrets here, just a tried and tested formula that works. So if you're looking to get rid of your central obesity, then you know now what you need to do.

I must warn you of something though. It's important for you to understand that your road toward achieving this goal is not going to be undemanding, and you will more than likely have to go through a number of obstacles to get there.

But, what you need to always bear in mind is that you WILL reach your goals providing you are committed and just keep following the outlined path. And whatever you do, avoid searching for shortcuts because they don't exist, as I am sure you have realized by now!

I may have disappointed you with this chapter, by ruining your belief that spot reducing belly fat is possible. However, I hope that I have helped you get on the right track and understand what it is you 'really' need to do in order to fight the flab!

8. GENES DETERMINES YOUR WEIGHT LOSS

Myth: If you come from a family that is overweight, it's much more likely that you will struggle keeping off the pounds, because your genes will always be against you!

Fact: Let me start by asking you following: Did you know that around 25% of your weight problem can attributed to your genes, and the remaining 75% is determined by your nutrition and lifestyle behavior?

In other words three quarters of your weight is governed by what you eat, how often you exercise, and whether you are prepared to work at maintaining a healthy, balanced lifestyle.

Only one quarter can be connected directly to your genes, so we can cast aside the genetic factor for being overweight. As you can see, the heritable issue does have some influence, but its role is minimal in comparison to the lifestyle aspect.

Genes are frequently used as a poor excuse to avoiding healthy living, and so many members of overweight families continue with the tradition of consuming an unhealthy diet.

This typically involves everything from hamburgers, coke, chips and whatever other sugary, salty stodge can be crammed into the shopping basket.

Folks think that if their genes are making them fat, then there's nothing they can do about it, and so go all-out on a lifetime eating binge.

It saddens me when I hear people say things like:

"Well, it's not my fault I'm overweight; it's my genes. Almost everyone in my family is fat because of genetics".

Know now that this is total nonsense, and that you are in much more control than you realize.

I understand that some people put on weight easier than others, and they also have to work a little harder at losing the pounds.

Even so, unless you have a medical condition that is causing you to be fat, and stay that way, then you can get your weight down. It is crucial that you are constructively self-critical. You might want to start by looking at yourself in the mirror and asking:

"Have I really done everything within my power to keep my metabolism as high as possible?" If you can't honestly answer that with a resounding "YES" then you need to reflect on "where you could make some improvements and get yourself into maximum gear.

When I was a lot younger, I used to hang around with this friend who claimed that his genes were a total disaster, and how they messed with his metabolism. He'd say that this was why he could never lose weight no matter how hard he tried.

He was so convinced about this that even his entire family were repeating the same phrase over and over again (just like a pandemonium of parrots), blaming family genes for his weight problem.

I really sympathized with him, and at that time I almost believed in his unfortunate dilemma. That was until I found out that he regularly dropped by at a local hamburger joint ordering the biggest item on the menu (with extra fries).

When I confronted him he said that there was little point at attempting to lose weight because of the gene issue, something proven by looking at his own family, where everyone was overweight. Little did he know that his real problem wasn't genetics at all, but the sheer amounts of junk food he consumed.

I happen to know that he is still grossly overweight to this day, and unfortunately he's developed several health disorders in recent times because of his obesity. His inability to be honest with himself has in fact caused him health concerns that could have been totally preventable.

Yet despite it all, he hasn't made any major lifestyle changes in an attempt to improve his health and general wellbeing. Sadly, cases such as this are far from unique.

If you can identify with any of the above, and you too blame your weight on your genes, then perhaps you might want to now reconsider your options. Don't be like my old friend, be different, and make a better life for yourself, starting today.

9. FAT IS REALLY HARMFUL TO HEALTH. ISN'T IT?

Myth: All fats are bad, and if you want to lose weight then you need to eat less of it!

Fact: There is a huge difference between the different types of fats, and although some are very harmful there are others that are not only healthy and necessary as part of a well-balanced diet, but they can actually contribute to weight loss, and help your body to function better, which in turn makes you feel great.

I admit it sounds strange, and I too had a hard time believing it when I first began researching diet and nutrition.

However, once I found credible evidence to back this up, I was soon able to identify the different fats, i.e., the good from the bad.

This meant I could eat healthier, and maintain my ideal weight easier. When it comes to controlling body fat, education really is the key.

Saturated & Trans Fats

These are the types of fats that you should avoid as much as possible. Unfortunately they are also the ones that are usually associated with a lot of the foods we consume in our daily meals, and that makes avoiding them pretty difficult.

The vast consumption of trans-fat has transpired as a result of modern society and the types of foods we've come to love.

You will find them in baked goods, breakfast cereals, energy bars (various), chips and crackers, cookies, candy, fast foods, frozen foods (TV dinners, pies, pizzas etc.), most packaged foods, soups (various), toppings and dips (various), and many other types of foods that are made by using partially hydrogenated oils. [9].

Saturated fats have been around since the dawn of time. These can be found in foods from animals, i.e., fish oil (especially menhaden and sardine), processed meats, red meats, rendered animal fats, butter, cheese, and whipped cream to name but a few.

Saturated fats can also be found in various plants, including; dried coconut, hydrogenated oils (palm, coconut), nuts and seeds (namely pili nuts, brazil nuts, macadamia), and various other plants [10].

Monounsaturated Fat & Polyunsaturated Fat

Now that you know what type of fats you should avoid at all costs, or at least as much as possible, let us now look at what the healthy fats are, and where we can find them!

These are the fats you should strive to include in your daily diet, and are the ones which can help you lose weight.

Although these names sound more like something you would find in nuclear physics, they are actually pretty simple to understand, and the main difference between the two lies in their chemical structure.

You can find monounsaturated fats in various vegetable oils such as olive oil, peanut oil, and sunflower oil.

Avocados and different types of nuts are also known to contain high amount of Monounsaturated fats [10].

Polyunsaturated fats are found in some types of fish, seafood, and oils like olive. Nuts are also known to contain high amount of polyunsaturated fats, especially walnuts and Brazil nuts [11].

According to the National Cholesterol Education Program (NCEP), you should try to maintain a diet that consists of around 10% polyunsaturated fats and 20% of monounsaturated fats in your daily food intake [12].

I know this might all sound easier said than done, but once you become more familiar with healthy foods, then eating well-balanced meals will become second nature to you.

So to recap this chapter; you have learned that there are good fats and bad fats, and that saturated & trans-fats are the ones to avoid as much as possible, whereas the monounsaturated and polyunsaturated fats are those which you should try to include in your diet.

Next time someone claims that all fat is bad, just show them this chapter!

10. VEGETARIAN DIETS ARE BETTER FOR LOSING WEIGHT

Myth: Vegetarian, or plant based diets, is the most efficient way to lose and maintain a healthy weight. This is because they tend to contain less calories and fat.

Also, people who are vegetarian are thinner than those who are not, which means that eating the same foods as they do will make you a leaner person too.

Fact: There are several studies that show a correlation between a vegetarian diet and weight loss.

However, there are no actual guarantees that following a specific vegetarian eating plan makes you lose more weight compared to a regular diet that is balanced with animal produce.

A study published in the International Journal of Obesity (IJO), showed that overweight adults who were instructed to follow a vegetarian diet for a period of 18 months, lost about 7.9% - on average - of their total body weight.

At the same time, a second group of adults within the same weight range were instructed to follow a regular diet.

The results showed that these participants lost, on average, 0.1% more weight than the group that followed the vegetarian diet. [13].

As you can see, the adults who consumed a regular diet actually lost slightly more weight when compared to those that were on the vegetarian program. Although vegetarians in general tend to be healthier and leaner than meat eaters, there could be other reasons for this.

According to Katherine Zeratsky, R.D., L.D., the key to losing weight is not a simple case of switching to a plant based diet.

You can still gain weight by consuming only vegetarian meals if you are not paying attention to the size of your portions, and type of foods you consume.

She also says that the reasons why many vegetarians tend to be leaner than folks who consume meats, eggs, and dairy products in their regular meals, is because the vegetarian diets usually contain less saturated fat.

In addition to this, those who know how to eat vegetarian meals correctly, have a sharp focus on consuming more fresh vegetables, fruits and protein derived from plants [14].

There are or course, many types of vegetarian, but here I am referring to those who eat a strict plant-based diet only.

My opinion is that anyone who is serious about eating healthy, well-balanced meals, need to start by evaluating their own current eating habits.

Taking inventory of your foods is a far better way to establish a tailor-made eating plan than trying to find a specific diet that is supposed to guide you towards healthier meals.

You need to get to know your own body, be mindful of how much and how often you consume food, snack in between, and of course the exact types of meals you consume in a typical day, week, and month.

For example, imagine that you are on a healthy vegetarian diet, yet you are still eating fried foods (plants as opposed to meats), and you frequently include treats such as cookies, milk chocolates, and other calorie bombs that quench your sugar cravings for a short time.

Such a way of eating will mean that no diet in the world can help you because you have not done away with the main culprit, which is consuming those foods that are full of calories filled with empty energy.

So unless you reeducate your palate and mindset completely, then the problem of weight will stay with you till the end, be you a meat eater or a vegetarian.

If you eliminate the main problem, I am convinced that you will lose weight no matter what type of diet you follow.

Cutting ties with old habits is never easy, but if you stop fighting AGAINST cravings and start fighting FOR a healthier lifestyle, then you're destined for success.

11. PRODUCTS LABELED AS 'ZERO TRANS-FAT'

Myth: If a product states "zero trans-fat" then there are no such fats contained within!

Fact: Trans-fat is known to be harmful to your heart. It raises your bad cholesterol (LDL), while lowering your good cholesterol (HDL). High LDL contributes towards cardiovascular diseases, including heart attack.

Trans-fat is often considered to be the worst type of the fat available for human consumption. Although most of us are aware of this fact, that doesn't simply mean we can cut it out of our diet by making a simple decision.

The problem with trans-fat is that it's almost impossible to avoid, especially if you've got other things to be getting on with than shopping in health stores and spending all day in the kitchen micro-analyzing every ingredient of every meal you prepare. [15].

So although we are more aware of the existence of trans-fat in food, we are still lured to eat it (unknowingly at times), because manufacturers employ all kind of shady tricks and clever marketing tactics as they include trans-fat into their products.

If you are someone who likes to read the nutritional facts on food labeling, and find an item that shows there is no trans-fat inside, or even states there is zero trans-fat included in the product, then you would have no reason to dispute it – right?

Wrong!

This is another food myth, or should that read as a 'legal con' perhaps?

Why?

Because the truth is that a product can contain trans-fat, but it doesn't have to be stated on the labeling like some other ingredients do.

So how can this be legal? Well, there are laws that regulate what can and should be on a nutritional label. According to the Food and Drug Administration (FDA), products can be labeled as zero trans-fat if they contain less than 0.5 g per item.

However, sometimes the phrase "trans-fat" is not used at all, but this doesn't necessarily mean the food item is free of it. There are ways you can quickly ascertain whether or not there is trans-fat inside the item by learning how to read the labels.

So, if you want to check for hidden trans-fat you can do so by interpreting words that are often used as synonyms for the term. These include:

- Partially hydrogenated oil
- Hydrogenated margarines
- Partially hydrogenated

That's pretty sneaky marketing going on there, and the majority of lay shoppers will not know about this ploy!

As you can see, the word "hydrogenated" is used in combination with some other term. This is just a clever way to camouflage the existence of trans-fat on the nutrition label attached to the product.

The strategy I use personally to avoid trans-fat - as much as possible - is pretty straightforward and simple. Firstly, I circumvent all temptation to consume any kind of fast food, junk food, or convenience foods, and whatever other terms are used to describe the same unhealthy nosh.

In addition, I cook my own meals whenever possible, always making sure to use only fresh groceries and steer well clear of adding any processed "ready to eat" items into my diet.

By following this simple suggestion, you too will drastically minimize your intake of trans-fat to a bare minimum, because it will be much harder for it to slip into your daily meals without your knowing.

I would also suggest you read the labels on each product before you put it into your shopping basket, making sure to take heed of the sneaky tactics to disguise trans-fat that I mentioned above.

I know that this all takes time, but you will soon become familiar with what to look out for, and before long you will be glancing at nutrition labels in nanoseconds.

And don't forget too, there will be many items that you purchase regularly, so once you know which ones are free of trans-fat, you will no longer need to read their labels anyway.

Remember, if you're the person that does the shopping, then you are the one who is responsible for identifying trans-fat in products you buy.

You have a responsibility to yourself and towards your family if you have one, because what you eat, is what they are going to be eating as well!

12. DAIRY PRODUCTS MAKES YOU FAT

Myth: The regular consumption of dairy products in your daily diet is going to make you fat and gain more weight over time – not lose it!

Fact: Dairy products are not fattening, and what's more is that they can have an opposite effect which has been proven through several studies.

But, before I tell you about these findings, I just want to let you know that I have been drinking milk, eating cottage cheese, and enjoying yoghurts, ever since I was a kid.

Today, I still have a solid body sculpture, and as I mentioned earlier, I also have a six pack to boot.

I don't say this to boast, but merely to convince you about the importance of including some dairy products into your regular diet, and to quash the myth that they should be avoided if you are to lose weight.

Because there is so much negative material out there regarding dairy products, you may still be unconvinced by my statements and assumptions, so I will try to assure you with two interesting studies on this very topic, after which I am sure will have changed your mind about this.

The first study, and the one I found most interesting, was published in the International Journal of Obesity, where 14 clinical trials experimented on 883 adults in the age range of 18-85. The idea behind the research was to see how dairy products affected the participant's weight, muscles mass, and fat.

Researchers found that 3-4 servings of dairy products - combined with a low calorie diet – actually contributed to weight loss when compared to those adults who completely skipped all forms of dairy produce from their daily diet [16].

The second study I found on this topic was conducted by Danit R. Shahar, RD, PhD. He concluded that calcium and Vitamin D (both of which are found in dairy products), may contribute to a healthy weight loss regime.

He studied 322 obese adults in their middle age, and found that those with highest calcium intake had lost the most weight overall.

It should also be noted that patients were not instructed to use a specific diet or workout routine during the course of the study [17].

Take cottage cheese example. It's known to be very low in fat yet contains a lot of protein which will fills you up.

This contributes to a better controlled weight loss plan by curbing hunger through the consumption of small amounts. In fact, many of the popular diets use cottage cheese in their meal planning.

Honestly, dairy produce has been a popular ingredient in our food since the very beginning of humankind, so claiming that it is responsible for making us all fat now, doesn't make any sense at all, especially when our society is dominated by so much processed and fast food.

The global obesity epidemic is a relatively new phenomenon, and we were all consuming dairy products long before entire nations got to be as fat as they are today.

There really is a lot of claptrap out there, and being able to separate the fact from the fabrication is the key to effective weight loss and sustainable weight maintenance.

Hopefully by now, I've managed to convince you to eat dairy products that are low in calories, and to only avoid those with a high fat content of say 5% or more. Follow these simple suggestions and you will not need to question the "dairy is bad for you" issue ever again.

Best of all, dairy will become a part of your well-balanced diet, and contribute towards shedding any unwanted pounds, while also helping to achieve long-term sustainable weight.

13. EGGS RAISE THE BAD
CHOLESTEROL LEVELS

Myth: It is recommended that we avoid eggs in our diet because they are known to raise bad cholesterol (LDL), which is acknowledged as a main contributor to cardiovascular diseases, and that includes heart attack.

Fact: The main reason why people buy into the idea that eggs raise bad cholesterol levels is because they contain the most cholesterol of all foods, or more specifically, the yolks do.

However, I have found studies that talk of the true benefits of eggs, so let's look at what they have to say about this.

Thomas Behrenbeck, M.D., Ph.D. states that cholesterol affects people differently and how much cholesterol you should consume in your daily diet depends on how healthy you are and whether you have any cardiovascular diseases.

Furthermore, Behrenbeck says that people should generally limit the amount of eggs they eat to just four per week, and those folks who want to eat a lot of them ought to remove the yolk, because that's where the high concentrations of cholesterol is found (1234mg per 100 grams) [18].

But, what if you want to eat eggs everyday – including the yokes - instead of just the recommended four per week?

Is this really so dangerous to health, or can you enjoy eggs daily without worrying about high cholesterol and an increased risk of heart diseases?

Well, I looked into this further and found a study led by Dr. Bruce Griffin who instructed 50 overweight individuals to consume two eggs per day during a 12 week period.

These volunteers were also given a specific low calorie diet to follow for the duration of the research.

At the same time, another group of individuals with the same characteristics as the ones above, were given the same low calorie diet, but there was a difference. This particular group was told that they could not consume any eggs at all during this 12 week period.

The collective results of this study were perhaps surprising, considering all the bad publicity we get about egg consumption. It was determined that both groups were able to lose weight but they also lowered their levels of bad cholesterol. There were NO significant differences in cholesterol levels found in either group [19].

So if both groups managed to lower their bad (LDL) cholesterol, even though 50 of them consumed two eggs per day, every day, for 12 weeks, then it shows that there is no real proof that eggs yolks increase the amount of bad cholesterol or the risk of heart disease.

I want to conclude by saying that the research and studies I've discovered, I found no concrete evidence that eggs actually cause bad cholesterol, and I firmly believe the main culprit for this is a sedentary lifestyle.

As someone who has always been fit and active, I never pay attention to the amount of eggs I consume on a daily basis.

I am completely convinced that by combing a healthy diet with regular exercise means I don't need concern myself about the amount of cholesterol found in eggs.

Almost every health issue related to weight derives more from an inactive lifestyle and poor diet. Eat well, eat in moderation, and become more active, is the real way to live, and those who don't are the ones who are sadly digging their grave with a knife and fork.

14. BANANAS ARE FATTENING

Myth: Don't eat bananas because they are full of carbohydrates and these are converted into fat inside your body!

Fact: This is actually one of my favorite myths because I've heard a whole variety of stories when it comes to bananas and weight gain.

The classic one is that bananas make you pile on the pounds because they are full of carbohydrates, which they are, but that doesn't mean you should exclude them. Does it?

What a lot of people don't get is that there's a huge difference between the two kinds of carbohydrates (see chapter six above), and while one type is linked to weight issues, namely the bad carbs found in white rice, and white bread etc., you should know that bananas contain fructose, which is one of the best carbohydrates you can eat.

Still not convinced?

All right, let's look at some studies that back me up on this. A study led by J.P Thakorlal and her team of researchers, found that green bananas might actually increase fat burning.

The resistant starch in green bananas simply prevents the body from using the carbohydrates as energy. Instead, Thakorlal and his team say that the human body is therefore compelled to burn the stored fat as energy, thus contributing to accelerated weight loss [20].

Sounds promising right, but these are green bananas, and they are not easy to eat because you need to cook them first, which is something many busy folks don't have time to do. And anyway, most of us just want to eat our tasty fruit immediately, as it's intended.

So, I wanted to find something that might prove regular, ripe bananas, can also be eaten without worrying about the weight issue. I researched a lot of sources and found exactly what I was looking for.

Martica Heaner, Ph.D., M.A., M.Ed. states in an article published on the reputable website, MSN Healthy Living, that a 'ripe banana' contains about 100 calories. That's fewer calories that most of the commercial sport drinks sold on the high street, and that makes it an ideal, and totally natural, sport snack.

She also points out that a ripe banana contains a lot of fructose, the fruit's natural sugar, when compared it to other fruits.

However, she emphasize that fructose is not in any way fattening (remember, it's a good carb). So now you know that yellow bananas are good for us [21].

I eat at least two bananas a day, one in the morning and one before my evening workout. One banana contains approximately 100 calories, which is the same as two regular sized apples or peaches.

Recently I have been waking up in the small hours of the morning feeling a tad hungry, so I eat one banana to curb my appetite before slipping back into bed.

I think this sudden late night hunger has something to do with intensifying my training sessions, but whatever the reason, the extra banana does the trick.

Although I don't recommend you grab a banana if you happen to wake up during the night (especially if you're not hungry), just bear in mind that if you ever do stir feeling famished, know that you can happily eat a banana without worrying about the weight myth associated with this fruit!

15. NUTS MAKE YOU FAT!

Myth: All nuts are known to contain a lot of fat and calories. That means if you consume them on a regular basis you run the risk of weight gain.

Fact: This is not a complete myth because nuts do contain a lot of calories and fat. However, that does not mean you should exclude nuts totally from your diet.

The key here is to consume them in controlled portions, and then you will find that most nuts will serve you very well indeed. They not only provide your body with essential nutrients, but can actually help with weight loss too.

Research conducted by McManus & Antinoro involved a study where they modified a weight loss diet by including a limited amount of foods that were rich in healthy fats. They compared the results with another group who were on a traditional low fat diet.

What they found was really very interesting. The group on the 'high in healthy fats diet' lost weight, whereas the ones on low fat diet actually gained 2.9 kg (6.2 lbs.), on average, over the duration of this 18 month study!

Researchers concluded the group that lost weight consumed fats found in nuts.

Their diet not only tasted better, but filled them up more, which made them stick to it religiously for the study period.

The group that gained weight was not quite so controlled or committed to the experiment, due mainly to their boredom with the traditional low fat diet [22].

According to Professor Rune Blomhoff (who specializes in nutrition, diet, and oxidative stress), and his team of scientist from the University of Oslo in Norway, consuming a handful of nuts (about 30g daily), is proven to help maintain a controlled weight and also helps towards lowering bad cholesterol [23]

So now you know that nuts are NOT fattening providing you don't overindulge and stick to the recommended daily portion of 30g.

It's important to mention though, that not all nuts are equal. So let us now look into the most optimal nuts from a health and weight management perspective.

The top 3 you should opt for are:

- Almonds,
- Peanuts
- Walnuts.

These are well known to have a positive effect on preventing cardiovascular diseases by keeping your blood vessels clean while decreasing the level of bad cholesterol.

There is a word of warning here though, and that is nuts are only to going provide you with all their nutrition in the raw form. In other words, avoid those which have been roasted, salted, or flavored with any other additives.

The Wonderful Walnuts

Another interesting fact worth mentioning is that walnuts are rich in alpha-linolenic acid, and are the only nuts that contain a significant amount of it. Alpha-linolenic acid is the omega-3 fatty acids found in various vegetable products, and are vital for normal metabolism [24].

Personally, I consume a few too many nuts. I have them at breakfast, lunch, and dinner as well. I am also a lover of big of milkshakes, and I always like to enjoy these with nuts too. I know my body well though, and that means I'm able to compensate this overindulgence in some other way.

I urge you to add the recommended portion of nuts to your daily diet. As you have learned here, a handful is more than sufficient to cater for you daily needs.

Perhaps the best thing of all is that they make great nutritional snacks, giving you an energy boost, while at the same time curbing hunger!

So next time you're chilling out watching that movie, forget the usual popcorn, bags of chips, and tasty dips, and choose nuts instead.

While they might not taste quite as good, just know that they're doing you good, which is more than can be said for the usual health-damaging munchies.

16. YOU SHOULD AVOID MEAT

Myth: Eating meat is not a good way for you to keep yourself healthy. Furthermore, it makes weight loss, and maintaining weight, difficult.

Fact: I must say that this is a myth that always gives me a good laugh. It goes against everything I've learned about successful weight loss and the body's ability to burn fat.

Meat is one of the best foods you can consume in order to stay healthy and control your weight, although there is one specific type of meat I recommend you avoid (more on this later).

In a study, led by Dr. Alfons Ramel at the University of Iceland, along with his team of scientists, studied groups of similar individuals where they were given protein from different sources. These groups were divided as follows:

- **Group A** - The individuals in this group were given lean meat as their primary source of protein.

- **Group B** - The partakers in group B were given cod (a low fat fish), three days a week as their primary source of protein.

- **Group C** - This group consumed cod five days a

week as their primary source of protein intake.

A common factor for all three of these groups was that they were to follow a strict diet during an eight week period. The results were interesting. Group C (the ones eating cod five days a week), lost the most weight overall and reached a noticeable reduction in fat mass [25].

It is also important to note that the individuals participating in this study were not on a high protein diet. Instead, only 17% of their total caloric intake daily came from protein, 35% from fat, and almost half of the calories (48%) from carbohydrates.

The conclusion we can conduct from the study above is that meat is not fattening or insalubrious; instead it can contribute to a healthy weight loss and also help to lower the amount of fat stored in the body.

I consume meat in my daily diet, always have done, and always will do.

But there is a specific type of meat I tend to avoid because of its high concentration of saturated fat, and as pointed our earlier, this is known to increase the level of bad LDL cholesterol.

The meat I am referring to is red meat, which is in my opinion not a healthy choice. Perhaps the most common red meats include:

- Beef
- Goat
- Lamb
- Pork
- Veal

VenisonI'm well aware of the various studies that say red meat is a good source of food and that it should be included in a well-balanced diet, but I don't agree!

There are far better, much healthier ways for us to get the protein, vitamins and minerals that are found in red meats.

Sure, it's great to have a tasty steak occasionally, but I will not include it, or any other red meats, as part of my regular diet.

I just care far too much about my health, especially when there are so many nutritious alternatives.

17. LIFTING WEIGHTS WILL BULK YOU UP

Myth: As a woman you need to avoid lifting weight because you can easily bulk up and gain pounds of unattractive looking muscles!

Fact: This is one of the myths I hear all the time when working out at my local gym. In most cases, the ones that really worry about this are women. It took me a while to convince my own wife that it's just a myth, and my goal with of this chapter is to do the same with you!

Picture this scenario; you've decided to lose some weight and your main goal is to get a leaner, firmer body.

After doing a little research, you then decide that it would be a good idea to get a gym membership as a way of getting started.

Now fully motivated, and having great expectations, you arrive at your first workout, but as soon as you enter the gym there is something that startles you.

As you look around, all you can see is a fitness center full of guys with pumped up muscles, resembling different versions of the Incredible HULK!

You're now asking yourself what on earth you are doing there, thinking that the gym membership wasn't such a good idea after all. It was certainly not your intention to end up looking like the Hulk!

Some of these guys were so bulked up they looked as though they'd explode if they got struck by a nail. You spend a few minutes checking the place out before leaving it, totally disappointed and utterly demotivated.

While this might sound like an extreme scenario, I have heard several people telling a similar story. I wanted to change this false perception so I needed someone to help me with my case study. I picked the person who was closest to me, my somewhat reluctant wife.

She was completely convinced that by lifting weights she would soon lose her womanly curves and feminine shape, and this is why she has always avoided them.

However, she was frequently complaining about how she wanted to get rid of the fat on the upper part of her arm, but didn't know how. Any exercises I suggested that used weights always fell on deaf ears – until now!

I decided to make a bet with her, and said that she will lift weights under my guidance for a period of one month and get the results she wants. If I failed to deliver, I promised to take care of all the laundry for a whole year.

She could not resist the bet regarding the laundry, and so decided to take me on with it, and we started with the training the very next day.

My wife complained all the time about how she would not like to get big arms, and constantly remarked on some of the other women at the gym that had the body of Tarzan.

I kept saying over and over that it's impossible to bulk up from lifting weights the way I'm instructing her, and that the inevitable 'muscle bulge' is one of the biggest myths when it comes to losing weight.

She wanted to quit many times but I kept encouraging her by reassuring her that the results she wants are just around the corner.

After just one month we evaluated the progress and she was really, really happy with what we had achieved. From then on, she was on cloud nine and you could see the happiness just by looking into her eyes. This is one bet, she didn't mind losing!

After just one month we evaluated the progress and she was really, really happy with what we had achieved. From that point on, she has on cloud nine and you could see the happiness just by looking into her eyes.

This is one wager, she didn't mind losing! I knew I would win the bet, because there was no way I was going to do all the laundry for an entire year.

More importantly, I was even happier to have convinced my wife about the importance of lifting weights to enhance her curves and shape. What we did was simply tone up, not bulk up, which are two completely different things.

Now, I want you to do the same as my wife did and try weights for one month. Make sure to give it your best and lift weights at least 3 times per week.

You might need an induction if you're new to this, so if you do, make sure you let one of the gym professionals know what it is you're trying to achieve. I then guaranteed you that you will get a stronger, leaner, and better-shaped body.

To summarize, you should know that the male hormone testosterone is required to build big muscles. Obviously men have much higher levels of this than women.

That means gaining big muscles or bulking up, while toning up, is impossible, unless you use some forbidden compounds and embark on intensive heavy weight training programs [26].

18. SKIP A MEAL OR TWO & LOSE WEIGHT

Myth: One of the greatest ways to lose weight quickly and efficiently is to skip a meal or two each day or at least on a regular basis.

Fact: Attempting to lose weight by skipping meals is like trying to swim wearing flippers made of lead. This is really a bad idea and whoever recommended it is talking through a whole in their head!

When it comes to various types of crash diets, most involve food depravation to some extent. They can be the most dangerous methods for losing weight, and remember, most of that weight loss is water anyway!

People who go on fast diets regularly, can, and do, cause themselves severe health problems, especially in the long term.

There are several studies that suggest those who skip breakfast and eat less than three times per day, you run the risk of being heavier compared to individuals who eat five to six times daily.

The rule of thumb here is to split your meals up so that you eat every three hours or so. Controlling your food intake in this way helps to suppress your appetite and keep your metabolism working.

I always have two fruits in my bag when going to work and I eat one three hours before lunch and the other one three hours after lunch.

This is a simple method of eating that really does help you to lose weight more effectively, and without depriving your body of the food it needs to function.

However, there is a drawback in that you will need a fair amount of discipline and determination in order to get positive results from this approach to controlled eating.

People who are new to the world of training and nutrition often believe that skipping meals is a kind of necessary punishment for being overweight, and that they deserve to be hungry for letting themselves go. It's the old 'No pain no gain' mindset.

A few years ago, a co-worker of mine who was (and still is) overweight, decided he wanted to get rid of his extra pounds once and for all. He simply skipped breakfast, lunch, and dinner, and limited his food intake to one apple and one banana each day. No easy feat for anyone, let alone someone who was used to eating big meals.

I still remember how he used to brag about how fast he was shedding weight, and the fact that his method was not only working, but working very well.

Despite what I told him, he still knew best, or so he thought, and told me that he was right, and I was wrong, and all I had to do was look at him to know that.

Depriving himself of food was no fun, but waking up and seeing his weight loss progress on the scales kept his motivation levels high.

In spite of this, he was still convinced that I was just talking gibberish and perhaps a little envious of his "success".

He even compared himself to me, and said that he was starting to get a six-pack just two weeks after beginning his fast diet, whereas I wasted a lot more time sculpturing my abs though my method of weight control and training.

But, as with everything in life, nothing lasts forever – good or bad - and in this particular case it turned out that I was right, and he was wrong after all. I knew this, but it took a wakeup call before he did.

A few days after this conversation on who knew best, I got a phone call from his mother. She told me that he was in hospital because his organs had stopped working normally.

It took him several months to recover completely from that crash diet, and he made a promise to himself, and the rest of his family, to never ever go on such a foolish eating regime again, no matter how desperate he was to lose weight.

To summarize this chapter, I want you to avoid anything that can be labeled as a fast, quick, or crash dieting. Although you might lose some pounds (mostly water weight though), you will gain the weight back really quick the moment you come off the diet.

Furthermore, you can cause disruption to the major organs inside your body, and depending on how much the diet interferes with their normal functioning, it could take quite some time to recover!

ABOUT THE AUTHOR

Mirsad writes all of his books in a unique style, constantly drawing connections between his past failures and the student's goals, so that you can avoid experiencing the same frustrations that he did. He doesn't promise you the world, but what he does promise you is that if you follow his tips and advice, you will reach your goals, guaranteed!

REFERENCES

1. Williams PT, Wood PD. The effects of changing exercise levels on weight and age-related weight gain. Int J Obes (Lond). 2006 Mar;30(3):543-51.

2. http://www.health.com/health/article/0,,20409933,00.html February 5, 2013

3.http://www.goodhousekeeping.com/product-reviews/research-institute/Good-Housekeeping-on-dr-oz Accessed February 5, 2013

4. Driver, H. S., & Taylor, S. R. (2000). Exercise and sleep. Sleep Medicine Reviews, 4, 387–402. doi: 10.1053/smrv.2000.0110

5. McArdle, W.D., Katch, F.I., & Katch, V.L. (2006). Essentials of Exercise Physiology. (3rd Ed.). Lippincott Williams & Wilkins: Baltimore, MD.

6. Academy of Nutrition and Dietetics Nutrition. Will Eating after 8 p.m. Cause Weight Gain? http://www.adaevidencelibrary.com/evidence.cfm?evidence_summary_id=250466. Accessed February 6, 2013.

7. Mehmet Cengiz Oz. Dr. Oz Busts Diet Myths, Pt 3 [Video File]. http://www.doctoroz.com/videos/dr-oz-busts-diet-myths-pt-3 Accessed February 6, 2013

8. Bossco C, et al. (2000). Monitoring strength training: neuromuscular and hormonal profile. Med. & Sci. in Sports and Exer. 32:202-208.

9.Trans Fat Now Listed With Saturated Fat and Cholesterol http://www.fda.gov/Food/ResourcesForYou/Consumers/NFLPM/ucm274590.htm Accessed February 1, 2013.

10. American heart Associaton. Know Your Fats http://www.heart.org/HEARTORG/Conditions/Cholesterol/PreventionTreatmentofHighC holesterol/Know-Your-Fats_UCM_305628_Article.jsp Accessed February 6, 2013.

11. State Governement of Victoria. Fats and Oils.

http://www.betterhealth.vic.gov.au/bhcv2/bhcarticles.nsf/pages/Fats_and_oils February 6, 2013.

12. Third Report of the National Cholesterol Education Program (NCEP) Expert Panel on Detection, Evaluation, and Treatment of High Blood Cholesterol in Adults (PDF), July 2004, The National Institutes of Health: The National Heart, Lung, and Blood Institute.

13. Burke LE, Warziski M, Styn MA, Music E, Hudson AG, Sereika SM. A randomized clinical trial of a standard versus vegetarian diet for weigh loss: the impact of treatment preference Int J Obes (Lond). 2008 Jan;32(1):166-76.

14. Katherine Zeratsky, R.D., L.D. http://www.mayoclinic.com/health/vegetarian-diet/AN01580 Accessed February 7, 2013

15. Abargouei AS et al. Effect of dairy consumption on weight and body composition in adults: a systematic review and meta-analysis of randomized controlled clinical trials. Int J Obesity 2012:1-9; Online: doi:10.1038/ijo.2011.269.

16. Shahar DR. Dairy calcium intake, serum vitamin D, and successful weight loss. Amer Jou Clin Nutr 2010. Published online ahead of print, doi: 10.3945/ajcn.2010.29355

17. http://www.mayoclinic.com/health/cholesterol/HQ00608 Accessed February 7, 2013

18. Gray, J., & Griffin, B. (2009). Eggs and dietary cholesterol – dispelling the myth. British Nutrition Foundation Nutrition Bulletin, 34, 66–70.

19. J Thakorlal, C O Perera, B Smith, L Englberger, A Lorens . Resistant starch in Micronesian banana cultivars offers health benefits. Pac Health Dialog. 2010 Apr;16(1):49-59. PMID: 20968236

20. http://healthyliving.msn.com/health-wellness/martica-heaner-phd-ma-med-1 Accessed February 8, 2013

21. McManus, K., L. Antinoro, F. Sacks. A randomized controlled trial of a moderate fat, low energy diet compared with a low fat, low energy diet for weight loss in overweight adults Int J Obesity 2001;25: 1503-11

22. Sabaté J. Nut consumption and body weight. Am J Clin Nutr 2003 Sep;78(3 Suppl):647S-650S 6. Fraser GE, Bennett HW, Jaceldo KB, Sabate J. Effect on body weight of a free 76 Kilojoule (320 calorie) daily supplement of almonds for six months. J Am Coll Nutr 2002 Jun;21(3):275-83

23. Blomhoff R. et al. Health benefits of nuts: potential role of antioxidants. Brit J Nutr 2007;96(SupplS2):S52-S60

24. Ramel A, Jonsdottir MT, Thorsdottir I. Consumption of cod and weight loss in young overweight and obese adults on an energy reduced diet for 8-weeks. Nutrition, Metabolism, and Cardiovascular Diseases, 2009; 9(10):690-696.

25. "Nutrition, Metabolism, and Cardiovascular Diseases"; Consumption of Cod and Weight Loss in Young Overweight and Obese Adults on an Energy Reduced Diet for 8-weeks; Alfons Ramel, Ph.D.; M.T. Jonsdottir; Inga Thorsdottir, Ph.D; Dec. 2009

26. Bossco C, et al. (2000). Monitoring strength training: neuromuscular and hormonal profile. Med. & Sci. in Sports and Exer. 32:202-208.

www.ingramcontent.com/pod-product-compliance
Lightning Source LLC
Chambersburg PA
CBHW070957290526
45795CB00005B/1682